The
Raw Crunch
Diet

"Strengthening your Body

from the Inside-Out"

Kathy Feldman

Published by SSI, Inc.

SSI, Inc. , 880 Holcomb Bridge Road, Roswell, Georgia 30076, U.S.A.
SSI Publishing, Inc. (Puerto Rico), 208 Ponce de Leon Avenue,
Suite 1800, Hato Rey , Puerto Rico 00918-1009

SSI, Inc., Registered Offices: Hato Rey , Puerto Rico 00918-1009

First Edition Printing, May 2005

Copyright © Kathy Feldman, 2005
LIBRARY OF CONGRESS DATA
Feldman , Kathy
The Raw Crunch Diet
2001012345
1. Diet - Non-Fiction. 2. Health & Fitness - Non-
Fiction.   3. Lifestyle - Non-Fiction. 4. Food - Non-Fiction. 5.
Cookbooks - Non-Fiction. I. Title.

ISBN 1-932623-09-4

Printed in China by Sun Fung Offset Binding Co. Ltd.
Set in Adobe Garamond
Editor, Mel Clark
Cover Design by AlphaAdvertising
Cover & Inside Photos by Michael Church Photography

The
Raw Crunch
Diet

Kathy Feldman

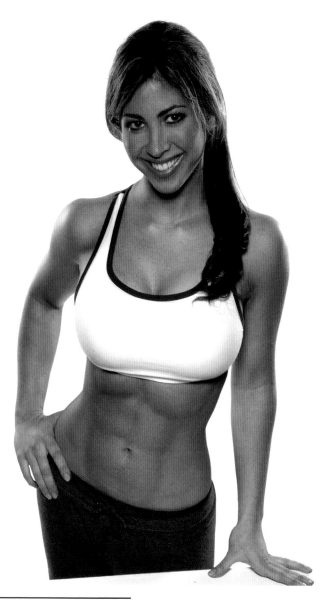

4   The Raw Crunch Diet

ONE

Hi, I'm Kathy, how's it goin'?

Let me guess, you'd like to spend less attention on your diet and more on your life? That's where I come in. For over a decade, I've devoted myself to this overwhelming search. *Why have I made this 12-year journey a full time job?*

Well, when you're a National Fitness Competitor, Model and Personal Trainer diagnosed and treated for extreme hypothyroidism (ultra low metabolism coupled with exhaustion, dry skin and excessive weight gain), you have to do something! It wasn't just for vanity sake either; my health was going down hill and fast. I've spent more time going the wrong route than the right, but at least I made it to this point successfully, cause I gotta good story to tell!

I've developed The *Raw Crunch Diet* based on my comprehensive and unique understanding of pure foods and true science. It involves dietary and lifestyle changes you can actually live with. No more counting calories, carbs, net carbs, fat grams, points, percentages, or precisely balanced meals.

See, my plan allows you to eat ANYTHING you want for dinner EVERY DAY OF YOUR LIFE! I mean that! Since the bulk of *The Raw Crunch Diet* is made up of raw, unprocessed fruits, veggies and nuts & seeds, which are so nourishing and cleansing, you can afford this luxury, without all the guilt. Your body does not have the added burden of trying to eliminate all the filth we eat and can run at optimal performance.

With a typical fad diet, you may look good on the outside for a few days (or weeks if you have enough willpower), but sadly even if the fad diet promoted weight loss, it's usually achieved at the expense of long-term nutritional health. When eating *The Raw Crunch Diet*, your body is fully nourished at the cellular level and it's reflected on the outside by a sleek physique and healthy hydrated skin.

G et ready to experience dramatic initial weight loss coupled by continued healthy fat loss. The initial weight loss comes mainly from the inflammation in your underlying tissues. I know it sounds a bit "out there" but this diet literally rinses your cells and clogged tissues clean. Oh yeah, my stubborn cellulite, GONE! This fat loss is not just temporary either, like those dreadful low-carb diets, so if you have bread at dinner, you won't blow back up like a water balloon. *"So what happens when I get off this Diet?*

T his will be the last time you'll ever ask that question. It's SO simple and SO satisfying! You'll learn to dismiss the myth that a healthy lifestyle means never eating a moist piece of cake again. No more worrying about food constantly, you'll finally enjoy eating! Your friends and family won't even realize your diet has changed; they will just be dying to know why you're lookin' so darn good.

TWO

What's the problem with obesity today?

Americans are just NUTRITIONALLY STARVED! Eating more food doesn't necessarily mean getting more nutrients. Believe it or not, overweight people are generally malnourished.

After consuming a typical meal or snack, your stomach feels full, while your body craves nutrients. You see, chances are that meal was unhealthfully processed. An example of processed food would be a typical junk food like a Danish; you can't just go out to your garden and pick a Danish off the vine, so therefore the Danish has been processed. White bread is less processed than a Danish, but still unhealthfully processed. You can go out to a field and harvest whole wheat berries, but when the fiber, most of the vitamins, minerals, fatty acids, and nutritional value is striped away when making white flour; when a token few synthetic vitamins and minerals are added back; when artificial flavors, chemical preservatives, and unhealthful oils are added you are definitely talking about a highly processed food! The same goes for white, refined sugar. Fresh whole fruit, on the other hand, which naturally contains sugar yet also contains a whole lot of nutrients (including fiber, which slows the absorption of sugar), is NOT a processed food. You get the idea.

Processed food is food that has been drastically altered from its natural state. These fake foods distort your appetite too. It's hard for you to exceed your caloric requirements with fruits and veggies because of the bulk and satiety you get from these foods, but over-eating unhealthfully processed foods like an entire bag of chips is no problem for some.

To further reduce their nutritional value most processed foods are cooked. When foods are overcooked much of their vitamins and minerals are damaged, or destroyed by heat, as well as their fiber. To make up for this, food manufacturers add nutrients back into the food, except these added vitamins & minerals are replicated in a lab.

I'm sure you've seen the long list of vitamins and minerals on an unhealthfully processed box of cereal or carton of concentrated orange juice labeled "with calcium". Adding individual vitamins or minerals can create imbalances with other nutritional factors in our body. The reason why nutrients are packaged the way they are in nature is because they require other nutrients in order to work properly in our body. That's why they say to take your vitamins with food.

Can you imagine how foreign a single vitamin tablet is to your body? They call these added vitamins and minerals *supplements*. Just think of the word "supplement". You are "supplementing" your diet with something you are not getting enough of through whole food. For people who do not eat well, supplements will not make up for that any better than "devoid of life" *energy pills* make up for lack of sleep.

Despite all of the modern advances, the best source of nutrients by far is whole food! It's always better to correct your diet, than to supplement it. The ideal purpose of *The Raw Crunch Diet* is to supply all the vitamins, minerals and nutrients one needs naturally in a readily available form enabling your body to function optimally without additional chemical supplements.

THREE

Okay, let's start with breakfast.

I know, you're not really hungry in the morning, plus you don't have the time. Hey, that's fine. There's a reason why your body isn't hungry when you wake up. Your body is smarter than you think. Why force concentrated foods into your system. "*Hey, but all the other weight loss books tell me that a big breakfast is critical.*"

Just listen. The word breakfast means, "*breaking a fast*". A *fast* is an extended period without food. Last night, you hopefully slept a good eight hours . . . yeah right? Well for those eight hours or about that, your body went without food. That's considered a *short fast*. When you woke up from that eight-hour sleep and ate breakfast, the *fast* was broken. In the human body, *fasts* are used to give your digestive system a break so that your body can devote its energy to cleansing and rebuilding.

Problem is, in this day and age our bodies are so run down by excess food and processed junk, that our typical *nightly fast* is not nearly enough time for the body to digest all the food from the previous day. Plus your digestive system slows down at night; it would probably like a little *"shut eye"* too. Instead, that 8-hour *fast* is solely devoted toward digestion, rather than cleansing.

Because of the unnatural cooked and over processed foods we eat, each meal leaves our digestive system sluggish and filled with toxic residue to deal with. We expect it to just cleanse and heal itself, but it has no time! The next morning, we just pour undigested food on top of the half-digested food still waiting there. Have you ever gorged yourself at dinner and still felt full the next morning? See what I mean. Over the past thousands of years, our bodies haven't changed much, but our diets have . . . drastically.

A light morning meal will help rid the body of these accumulated toxins and restore itself back to health. This morning cleansing process is a VERY CRITICAL part of *The Raw Crunch Diet.* Our digestive system needs this short, well-deserved rest in the morning. It will renew your ability to maintain optimum health.

FOUR

I'm going to explain your light morning meal

in a second . . .

I just need to throw in a quick biology lesson first. I promise to make this painless.

After food enters the stomach it travels into the small intestine (we have around *twenty-five feet* of small intestines for the slow absorption of plant food), food then enters the large intestine and continues through the colon (which makes up the majority of the large intestine) until the solid waste is finally excreted. Most people on the Standard American Diet (SAD) experience transit times of *seventy-two hours* or more. That means dinner last night could be chilling in your colon for days. In fact, upwards of eight (8) meals of undigested food and waste material could be sitting there, right now. The longer your body is clogged with *rotting food* in your colon, the greater the risk of developing various forms of illness. It's a breeding ground for bad bacteria.

As a natural secretion to protect the surface of your colon's membrane, the body creates mucus, trapping toxins to escort them out of your body. Dairy products, animal protein, processed foods, coffee and alcohol create the most mucus and congestion (since fruits and veggies are not foreign to the body, they don't cause much secretion of this sticky mucus). After years of *bad eating habits* this thick mucus begins building up and lines the colon (like a clogged bathroom sink waiting for a "drano cleanse").

Thank goodness your colon can stretch to five times its diameter; otherwise our colon could be blocked completely by this mess. Unfortunately, water and some minerals must also be absorbed in the colon. Yet this mucus build-up inhibits proper absorption of nutrients and water, as well as slowing our *normal peristalsis* (uh oh, big word there, sorry).

See, your colon is lined with these muscles that contract and send waste through to be excreted, that's all *peristalsis* means. If those muscles are slowed-down so is your systems transit time and because of that, wastes just sit there rotting.

Good news though, *The Raw Crunch Diet* dramatically decreases the *transit time of waste* matter avoiding toxic buildup. Besides, as you consume more raw fruits, veggies, nuts and seeds as a staple part of your diet, your body is finally nutritionally satisfied, properly hydrated and progressively it requires less food.

FIVE

So needless to say a light morning meal

is a good idea!

Here's how it works.

Remember, you want to keep your body in a cleansing mode as long as possible. When you wake in the morning I highly recommend an ultra cleansing, highly nutritious whole food superfood combination called *Vitamineral™Green.* Mix one tablespoon of *Vitamineral™ Green* with about four to six (4-6) ounces of your favorite juice. I'd prefer fresh juice, but do your best. *Vitamineral™ Green* is so highly concentrated with no bulky fillers like apple pectin, soy lecithin, whey, or rice bran and no stimulants or artificial sugars! Unlike incomplete, isolated multi-vitamin and mineral supplements, *Vitamineral™*

Green does not need to be taken with food because IT IS FOOD! These nutrients are all in the form of whole food green vegetables and superfoods such as whole leaf wheat grass, whole leaf barley grass, nettle leaf, shavegrass, oat grass juice, alfalfa leaf juice, broccoli juice, dandelion leaf juice, kale juice, spinach juice, Spirulina, Chlorella, burdock root, ginger root, nopal cactus, carob pod, Icelandic kelp and finally Nova Scotia dulse. *Vitamineral™ Green* does NOT have any isolated vitamins and minerals added to it. Naturally occurring in its botanical ingredients are all the major minerals (including calcium, magnesium, potassium, non-toxic plant iron, boron), all the B vitamins, a full spectrum of trace minerals, natural Vitamin C, soluble and insoluble fiber, complete protein, essential fatty acids, enzymes, hundreds of carotenoids, chlorophyll and tens of thousands of phytonutrients! YOUR BODY WAS DESIGNED TO RECOGNIZE THIS FORM OF NUTRITION. *Need I say more? This is some good stuff.*

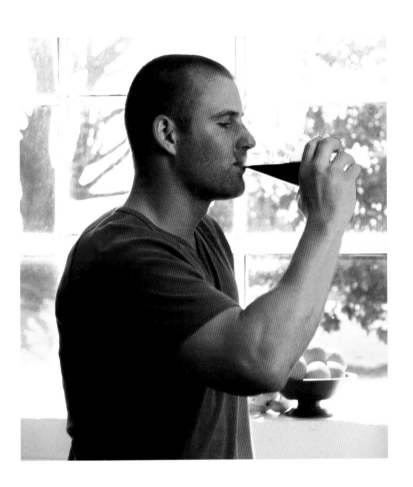

Hey, if my husband can drink his *Vitamineral*™
Green EVERYDAY, sometimes twice a day, SO
CAN YOU!

Next, have a glass of purified water (tap water is out because of all the chemicals and pollutants in it). And no, not that artificially sweetened, clear, carbonated, fruit flavored mess. That's not water, it's artificial and full of hard to digest chemicals.

Continue drinking water in the morning until you get hungry. Now it's time for fresh fruits. Any fruit, like apples, oranges, grapefruit, pineapple, peaches, pears, melon, grapes, berries, mangos, kiwi or whatever you like. Try to eat organically grown fruits in order to cut down on your exposure to toxic fertilizers, insecticides and herbicides.

Organic farming also produces more nutrient-rich soil, which nourishes the plants and therefore nourishes you. Organic products do cost more, but you should compromise something else in your budget, not YOUR HEALTH or the health of your environment. Even today's organically grown produce (although vastly superior to conventional produce) is still not nearly as nutritious as it once was. Plants begin to lose their vitality the moment they're harvested. During the approximately three weeks it takes for a fruit or vegetable to reach the plate of the consumer, some of its nutritional value will disappear. This is another reason why I recommend the *Vitamineral™ Green*. Consider it your daily dose of insurance.

Fresh produce is better than frozen, but frozen is far better than canned. When fruits or vegetables are canned, heat, additives, coloring, salt and sugar alter their original state. Dried fruit often contains added sugar and chemicals to give it a more appealing color and retain more water so producers can charge more money per pound. Regardless, dried fruit doesn't contain much water and bulk, so it's easy to overeat. Like I said before *"Fresh is best"*!

I like to have one type of fruit at a time to further ease digestion, but I'm pretty flexible here. Just think, any combination of fruit is far better than your previous diet. For instance, have one orange and if that's not enough, have another orange. Bananas are a bit denser fruit and great following a workout. Guys and athletes may need upwards of four (4) oranges or four (4) bananas in the morning, especially if they train in the morning. Listen to your body. This is not a cookie cutter diet. You have to mold it to meet your individual needs.

Your body's elimination cycle is the strongest between midnight and noon, so at least try to make it until noon on only *Vitamineral™ Green*, fresh fruit and water. So why only *Vitamineral™ Green*, fresh fruit and water? The *Vitamineral™ Green* and fresh fruit helps to keep your body in the cleansing mode, while providing natural bulk fiber that acts as a sweep through your colon. Remember, you always want to increase transit time. We don't want anything just hangin' out in our colon, right? We want to absorb the nutrients we need from the food and say goodbye. Since the fruit and *Vitamineral™ Green* help to loosen up old toxins in your colon, you'll need extra water to dilute them

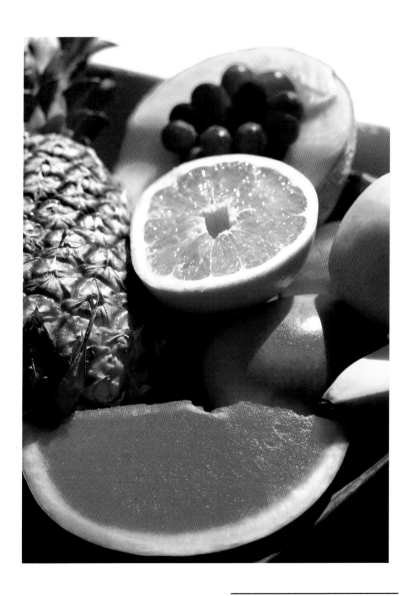

and flush them out. When your body is in a cleansing mode, you are also releasing toxins from your organs and tissues, which release into your bloodstream before they are excreted. If you don't have a lot of purified water in your system to dilute them, you could actually feel worse before you feel better. Fruits are a rich source of potassium, which also helps to remove accumulated fluids from your tissues. The water in fruits and veggies is "structured" water, which is the purest water you can drink. If you notice any detoxifying side effects like headaches or weak feelings, drink more water and if they persist, see your doctor. Guys should drink around a gallon of purified water a day and females should drink around three-quarters of a gallon per day, unless otherwise directed by your physician.

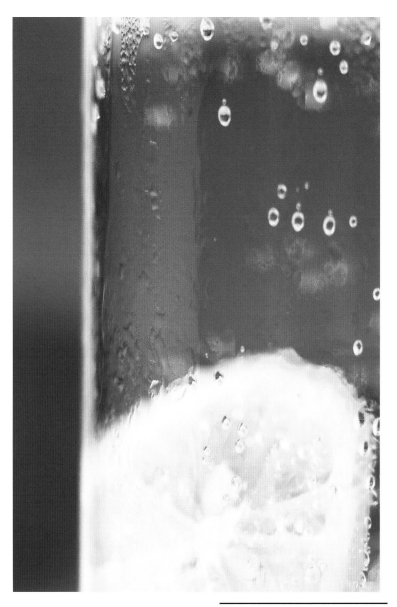

SIX

"Hey, Kathy, what about the acid in fruits?"

If you're one of those people who think fruit is too acidic on your stomach in the morning, keep this in mind, coffee, carbonated beverages, artificial sweeteners, meats and dairy products, *are much more acidic than alkaline fruits and vegetables* (even acidic lemons and limes have an alkalizing effect on the body when they are metabolized). As you can probably tell from these food examples, the average American diet is strongly acidic. Since our kidneys keep the acid/base concentrations of our blood constant, they have to work much harder to handle the acid load of the Standard American Diet (SAD). Our kidneys need a well-deserved rest in the morning too.

For those of you who have a sensitive stomach in the morning, drink a warm cup of water with a pinch of finely grated fresh ginger root and the juice of a quarter lemon slice. This is a perfect drink anytime of the day. *The ginger sooths your stomach and the lemon acts as a mild natural diuretic and laxative, stimulating digestion.*

This morning cleanse will keep your energy up like crazy and you won't believe your productivity. Energy is no longer wasted that was previously devoted to digestion. Your need for coffee will soon dissipate too. That's good because, coffee brings a halt to your morning cleanse faster than you can say, "low-fat sugar-free soymilk latte".

You can't disrupt your morning cleanse! I can't stress how important this is for fat loss! Green Tea is a great alternative beverage for coffee. Yes it contains caffeine, however, it also contains the amino acid, theanine, which is a caffeine antagonist and actually helps to balance the effects of caffeine. Green tea is much better than any other kind of caffeinated tea for this reason and of course far better for you than coffee.

Coffee actually drains your energy. It affects your blood sugar giving you a high followed by a deep low. This means your blood sugar is instantly elevated and then dropped considerably. Low blood sugar stimulates the appetite even if you have just eaten a full meal. No wonder a cream filled chocolate-coated donut with sprinkles tastes so good with a cup of coffee.

In fact, coffee also masks your need for sleep. By replacing your daily coffee with green tea, you will finally have the chance to feel what your body has been trying to convey to you all along and I suggest you listen. If you keep pushing your body the way you are, that body of yours is gonna age . . . fast.

Oh yeah, don't let me forget, if you're thinkin' you can get your energy boost from a soft drink instead, wrong, they contain loads of refined sugar AND caffeine, plus the carbonation makes it VERY acidic. No diet drinks either; artificial sweeteners are potent chemical replacements to sugar and they also effect your blood sugar, which increases your cravings. Have you noticed how you can eat more food when you have a diet soda with that meal? I sure have. You can't fool that body of yours.

You will soon realize that the cleaner and more naturally energized your body becomes, the more your body will try and reject coffee. Coffee will start to feel harsh and acidic on your stomach. Non-natural addictive drugs such as coffee, alcohol and cigarettes actually lose their appeal once the body is cleansed and balanced from *The Raw Crunch Diet.*

If a person is eating a more natural diet, caffeine and sugar have an even more disturbing effect on the system. For me, one cup of coffee has the effect of maybe four cups for you right now. My body has stopped protecting itself from the toxins of a modern diet, because it's in less contact with them. I also react strongly to alcohol. My husband calls me a "cheap date". Your tolerance will go down drastically too. And regardless of the advertising hype, "a six-pack does not equal a six-pack", but *whatever helps you sleep at night sweetie.* As dieters get smarter, so do the marketers.

SEVEN

"Oh, and what about those diet pills?"

Please promise me that you'll stay away from diet pills! Been there, done that, got a tee shirt. These pills speed up your *heart rate* and give you extreme energy highs and lows. But, your *heart* muscle never gets a chance to rest! Other muscles in the body that are tired and overworked can rejuvenate with sleep. Therefore, any damage you do to your *heart* now, will be there for the rest of your life.

Plus, something else, nothing you do to control your weight is more important than keeping your *liver* healthy. Your *liver's* main function is to filter toxins from your blood, so diet pills tax the *liver* since they are full of chemicals your body tries to reject. This distracts the *liver* from doing its second job of metabolizing FAT and SUGAR.

The minute you stop taking these pills, you'll pack the pounds right back on and then some. No one wants a sluggish *liver*. Rather than wearing your body down with weight loss pills, take my well worn advice and follow this nutrition plan to radiant wellness and permanent fat loss.

If you have abused diet pills or any other drugs like coffee, cigarettes, or alcohol you may want to use an awesome product I suggest called *Liver Rescue III+* to further assist your liver during this cleansing process. I know, I know, there are so many products out there these days to choose from, but the *Liver Rescue III+* and *Vitamineral™ Green* are the most highly effective nutritional products I've found, which work in conjunction with *The Raw Crunch Diet* to nourish your body COMPLETELY!

See, when the liver is toxic, it dumps toxins into your colon via bile. Then, if your colon is toxic (which almost everyones is prior to *The Raw Crunch Diet*) these toxins get reabsorbed into the blood stream and much of them are sent back to the liver and then back to the colon via bile and then back to the liver, etc. . . but to your advantage, *The Raw Crunch Diet* supports both colon and liver health.

EIGHT

Okay, sorry about that, let's get back on track . . .

So basically, *Breakfast* should be composed of *Vitamineral™ Green,* fresh fruits and lots of pure water. *But where is my protein, don't I need protein in the morning?*

Well, let's put it this way, most Americans suffer from a protein overdose, but you're right, fresh fruits don't contain much protein. However, Spirulina and Chlorella in your *Vitamineral™ Green* are the world's highest known sources of complete protein and they're easy to absorb and digest. Would you feel better if I suggested a *fat free* and *taste free* egg white omelet? Eggs are pretty unappetizing to humans unless they are cooked. . . wouldn't you agree? Cooking these animal proteins allows them to avoid our sensory safeguards that would normally *prevent us* from eating them. But hey, fry'em up and now they're edible. Cooking denatures their protein components, which leaves them harder to digest and utilize. Well, that counts them out in the morning. . . "harder to digest" is the last thing your worn out gut wants to hear!

So don't focus so much on protein in the morning, you're absorbing plenty of vital nutrients from *Vitamineral*™ *Green* and raw fruits. Plus, the combination of the fiber in the fruit, which you'll be eating pretty regularly throughout the morning combining with the *Vitamineral*™ *Green,* will keep your blood sugar stabilized and your belly happy.

NINE

It seems that everything you read these days tell you to "skimp-out" on CARBS.

The thing is your muscles are actually hungry for fast-absorbing carbohydrates, like fruit, rather than protein in the morning. See when you eat carbohydrates (like fruits and vegetables), they are converted to blood sugars and are stored mostly in your muscles as glycogen to be accessed for energy. Glycogen is just the technical term for *stored carbohydrates*. When you wake in the morning all of your glycogen reserves within your muscles have been depleted from your eight hour fast. In fact, blood sugar for proper *brain* function is also depleted. Protein is the last thing on your MIND, *it* needs fuel and so do your muscles.

Say you eat a high protein, low carb morning meal, your body will have to work much harder to transform some of that PROTEIN you eat into blood sugar or glycogen since this is the preferred fuel source of your *brain* and muscles. Converting protein to an energy source is very hard on your body. Why not make it easy on your body in the morning and eat natural carbohydrates that are easily converted to blood sugar, like fruits.

TEN

"But what about high protein diets, Kathy?"

Most high protein diets suggest that lean animal protein is "our most powerful ally when attempting *weight loss*" since it has twice the *thermic effect* of either fats or carbs. *Thermic effect* means that protein ingestion heats your body and helps you burn more calories than if you ate fruits, veggies, nuts and seeds. It does this because *animal protein is so much harder for your body to digest.*

Protein makes you feel full longer because *it sits in your gut trying desperately to breakdown.* Well yeah, sure your body burns more calories to break it down, but at the expense of your *kidneys, liver* and digestive health. Fiber (bulk) also makes you feel full longer on fewer calories, but it actually enhances healthy digestion.

When your body tries to break down animal protein in the gut, it generates *ammonia* which is extremely toxic, especially to the *liver and kidneys*. To protect itself from this toxic substance, your *liver* converts it to *urea*, which is less toxic than *ammonia*, but it's still a waste product and needs to be eliminated. Your *kidneys* remove *urea* from the bloodstream and eliminate it as urine.

Once again, this creates more stress on the *liver and kidneys*. It requires a large amount of water loss in the urine to dilute and flush these compounds from our body.

These high animal protein diets don't tell you to "drink like a fish", but they should with all this excess protein they're prescribing. But hey, you lose lots of weight on those diets, right? Yeah at first, by becoming dehydrated, making your next high protein meal even harder on your system. Because excess animal protein consumption produces an acid load on the *kidneys*, another problem is created. The body has to *neutralize the acid*. It does this by stealing vital alkaline minerals, like calcium, potassium and magnesium from the bloodstream, muscles and bones. *No wonder we need so much extra calcium these days.*

Raw plant foods are alkaline-based, not acidic. They not only prevent excess calcium loss; they also supply calcium to build strong bones while providing a good source of *clean burning* protein. *Clean burning* simply means, that raw plant foods release *only* carbon dioxide and water as by-products when they are converted to sugar, which causes very little digestive stress. As you can see, eliminating carbs from your diet and *replacing them with excess protein* is not only absurd it's dangerous. If you want to burn more total calories, while keeping your *liver, kidneys and digestive system* healthy and strong, just eat *The Raw Crunch Diet.* It's that simple!

ELEVEN

Let me fill you in on some basic secrets about our human system . . .

It's no coincidence that plant food contains just the right amount of protein to build and maintain the human body. Plant foods are where some of the strongest animals in the animal kingdom get their protein. Everyone thinks that it's close to impossible to build muscle without eating masses of animal flesh and protein powders, but check out the muscular physique of a horse. *Talk about horsepower!* Gorillas are vegetarians too and they could show us all up in the gym. Besides, ever looked at a tiger's teeth? How 'bout a horse's teeth. Now look at your own teeth. What do you think humans were designed to eat? Sure, meat is the staple of a tiger's diet, but our body's design and our nutritional requirements are very different from the tiger. Plus, their meat in the wild is raw and it's hasn't been contaminated with growth stimulants, hormones and antibiotics. When we look at other mammals in nature, we don't see any incidence of degenerative diseases. Hmm, wonder why? Our gut also has more trouble breaking down flesh for absorption in our twenty-five (25) feet of small intestines. On the other hand, raw meat eating animals have a much *shorter gut* for easy digestion. We are the only mammal in nature that cooks our meat, but understandably we have to do something to kill all that bacteria from our massively overcrowded animal production facilities. For all you strength-trainers out there worried about loosing muscle size, I assure you, if you have any muscle loss from this program, it won't be from lack of protein, just lack of steroids and growth hormones in all the excess meat that you were probably eating on your previous diet. I always thought that I was a "natural" fitness competitor. Prior to my fitness competitions, I always passed the lie detector tests as "drug free". Glad they didn't do a *blood test*, huh? I had all kinds of growth hormones and steroids in my system *just from the excess meat* I ate. I strongly believe that my typical six (6) (yes, six) high protein meals a day lead to my *thyroid hormone disorder* at such a young age. There are naturally so many hormones in meat *not to mention the "added hormones" in todays factory farmed meats* and *"hunny, you don't mess with a woman's hormones".* I'm leaner and more muscular now than ever before on *The Raw Crunch Diet.*

But what about fish, they say it's so good for you? Fish is actually a double-edged sword. Yes, it is one of the greatest sources of omega-3 essential fatty, which have endless health benefits, but when you cook omega-3 oils (like the ones in fish) they suffer the most damage of any other oil, releasing highly toxic chemicals. Despite the fact that fish does not have the immediate negative cardiovascular effects as other meats, fish still contains uric acid forming animal protein, which is very harsh on your system. Ocean or freshwater *wild fish* is potentally harmful too, considering that our waters are so much more polluted these days with industry run offs and other contaminants. Not to mention *farm raised fish* are packed in closed water systems and pumped with antibiotics to prevent disease. They are also usually fed a grain-based diet; therefore they obviously contain substantially less omega-3 fatty acids than *wild fish*. If you still plan to include *wild fish* in your *dinner meal of choice*, that's your indulgence. But not to worry, with all the other plant forms of essential fats in *The Raw Crunch Diet*, you'll get plenty of healthy fats!

TWELVE

"Hey, what about yogurt or some cereal in the morning, that's healthy, right?"

First off, we are the only mammals that drink another mammal's milk. Plus milk and milk products are cooked and processed, *so they stop the morning cleanse dead in its cow tracks.* Milk is mucus forming and contains growth hormones, steroids and antibiotics, so if you must have it, at least get organic forms and save it for your dinner meal.

I'm sure you've heard that yogurt is good for you because of all the friendly bacteria cultures it contains. See, your *colon* is home to good bacteria too, called probiotics, which help us to stay healthy and aid digestion. After the use of antibiotics, it is especially important to replenish these friendly cultures in your *colon*. That's because antibiotics not only kill the bad bacterial infection, they also disrupt the good bacteria in your *colon*. They're right. Yogurt does contain friendly bacteria cultures to replenish the *colon*. Unfortunately, yogurt is also processed with sugars or artificial sugars and probably more disguised antibiotics from its milk base, if it's not organic milk. BUT NOT TO WORRY, your *Vitamineral™ Green* includes a comprehensive probiotic mixture and in quantities far greater than you could ever get in yogurt.

And don't say, "I ONLY need probiotics after getting off antibiotics." Not if you eat any non-organic animal protein for dinner. Antibiotics are used as growth promoters in animal food production. Non-organic animal protein and over prescribed antibiotics are causing major forms of bacterial resistance in humans in our new 21st Century. So instead, feel free to add another serving of *Vitamineral™ Green* anytime you feel a cold coming on.

So no milk or yogurt? Where do I get my calcium from? You'll get plenty of calcium by adding calcium rich vegetables to your diet. Since animal protein consumption actually leaches needed calcium from your bones, reducing animal protein consumption will prevent further calcium loss.

So what about soy milk and soy yogurt? Yeah, it is a better choice than cow milk, but I prefer whole food soy products, rather than processed soy milk and soy yogurt. *Tempeh* (pronounced tem-pay) is made from organic whole soy beans. It tastes great and has a wonderful texture, not to mention it's high in clean-burning protein. But I'll come back to more *Tempeh* details around your lunch time.

Not all soy products are healthy though. If you read ingredient labels, you've probably seen soy protein isolate listed in all kinds of non-natural foods like cereals and protein bars. Soy protein isolate is used as a cheap way to add protein to foods in order to make them seem healthy. It's actually the left over by-product of creating soy oil. So instead of throwing it away, it gets added to processed foods for protein. The high temperature process used to create soy protein isolate also makes it difficult for our bodies to absorb the actual protein it offers. *The key is the quality of protein, not quantity of protein.*

In fact, there is no essential nutrient in meat or dairy that is not also available in fruits, vegetables, nuts and seeds and in a form that is much easier to digest. However, THERE ARE MANY ESSENTIAL NUTRIENTS THAT CAN ONLY BE GAINED FROM PLANTS.

Fruits & vegetables not only contain sustainable amounts of protein, carbohydrates and fat, they have them in the quality and proportions that are optimum for human health.

We're not talking the 40-30-30 ratios, like some

popular fad diets, we're talkin' *Mother Nature's* ratios. I don't have to teach your body to eat this way, it already knows and prefers it. It's your mind I have to convince.

THIRTEEN

Let's see now, we are only to about mid-morning in our meal plan . . .

Are you hungry yet? Yeah probably, since it's only been *Vitamineral™ Green,* fruit and water up until this point. Remember, fruits digest easily leaving the stomach quickly so you're probably experiencing an empty stomach about now. It's because we're so accustomed to eating concentrated foods these days, which are difficult to digest and stick to our stomach for hours. This light feeling you are experiencing may make you feel that you are not eating enough or getting enough nutrition.

Believe me *The Raw Crunch Diet* is infinitely superior to your old diet. You get more true nutrition out of one fresh organic orange than you can out of the standard American's full course meal. Besides, it's probably only noon and you've got plenty more time in your day for even more nourishment.

Speaking of nourishment, it's now time for that scrumptious *Raw Crunch® Bar*. These bars are not considered a supplement, like a "typical energy bar", protein powder, or vitamin. They contain only whole raw ingredients including: Organic Sesame Seeds, Organic Sunflower Seeds, Organic Flaxseeds, Organic Pumpkin Seeds, Organic Cashews, Organic Pecans, Organic Macadamia Nuts, Raw Honey and Celtic Sea Salt®. Currently they come with either: Organic Wild Blueberries, Organic Cranberries, Organic Dark Chocolate Chips, or Wild Crafted Goji Berries.

Remember, read ingredients carefully, that is, *if you can even pronounce them* and if you can't, chances are that it's a chemical your liver will have to work overtime to detoxify.

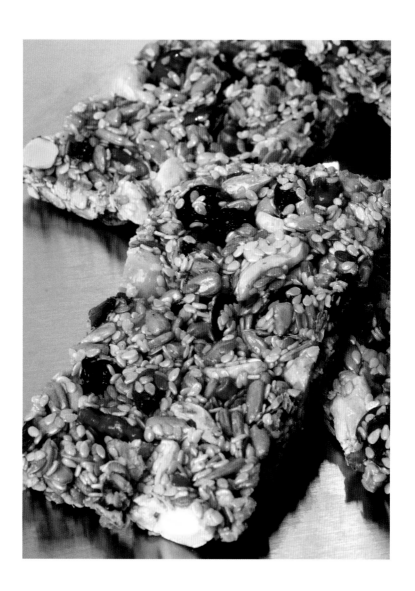

Raw Crunch® Bars are an uncooked, unprocessed, nutrition boost, free of artificial supplements, colors, flavorings and preservatives. They stabilize your blood sugar and are great for natural appetite control. By keeping your blood sugar stabilized, you are more likely to release stored body fat for energy. The hardest part for people to grasp is that you have to add *heart healthy fats* to your diet if you want to lose excess body fat. The healthy fats in these bars lean you up like crazy, while lubricating your joints, digestive tract and especially your skin.

Most cooked commercial energy bars, in addition to their unhealthy saturated fat, contain so much artificial sweeteners and cheap synthetic vitamins and protein that you're almost better off eating a candy bar. That's why my husband and I began making our own healthy bars. As athletes ourselves, we understand the value of a clean burning fuel for intense workouts, as well as a satisfying snack at the

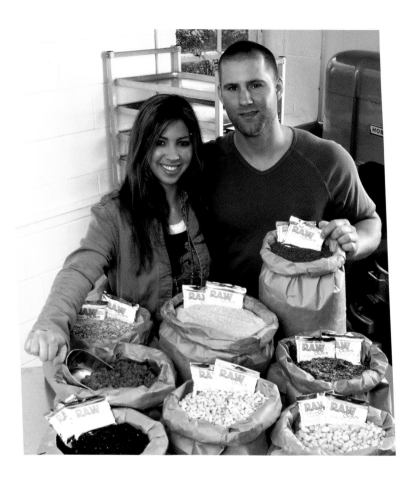

Here's my husband, Ross and I, in the facility where we *handmake* the *Raw Crunch® Bars.*

office. In the *Raw Crunch® Bars*, we formulated the most nutrient dense antioxidant rich raw ingredients.

If you were to look at a chart of prime food sources rated with every vitamin and mineral we know of, you would see nuts and seeds listed at the top. We then added berries and dark chocolate . . . ingredients that top the list of naturally occurring antioxidants. Although we use very little Raw Honey in our *Raw Crunch® Bars,* Raw Honey is not a refined sugar like "white sugar"; it is a sustaining energy source. This unique Raw Honey we use in our bars is harvested-by-hand and is intensely flavorful. Our *beekeepers* are passionate about the well-being of their *bees.* And the Celtic Sea Salt® we use contains a natural balance of sodium, magnesium and potassium, which regulates fluid balance in the body. With all of this in combination you're gonna be so healthy, you won't know what to do with yourself.

FOURTEEN

So let's get to that mid-day meal. . .

This meal should be a satisfying salad, but this salad is very easy to pre-make for work. Just throw in some mixed greens in a travel container. Toss in some carrots, cucumber, tomato, fresh sprouts, whatever veggies you like, and all you want! Sliced mangos, pears, apples, or grapes are also great additions. Now for the most important part, add some healthy raw fat. Avocados are an incredibly nutritious fruit and are an excellent source of healthy raw fat. I eat a whole avocado in my salad everyday. Guys and athletes can eat two whole avocados in their salad. If you don't like avocados do me a favor, just try it. If you still can't stand the taste, I tell ya what, I'll let you use two tablespoons of your FAVORITE salad dressing on your salad. Not the fat-free version either! Now will you eat it? Come on, avocados don't have much taste anyway. You need more substance here!

Just remember, the more healthy fats that you consume during the day from foods like avocados and *Raw Crunch® Bars*, the less calories that you will consume at your *dinner meal of choice*. These healthy fats will satisfy your hunger, thus reducing your appetite and lowering your total food consumption. Even though dietary fat contains more calories than protein or carbs, its effect on curbing appetite results in less daily calorie consumption. These healthy added fats give you energy, lean you up like crazy and make your skin vibrant and glowing as well as reduce digestive stress. Don't skimp out!

Cooking food destroys some of the nutrients, enzymes and fiber, however, some nutrients are actually better absorbed when they are lightly steamed, like those in asparagus, green beans, squash, broccoli, spinach, brussel

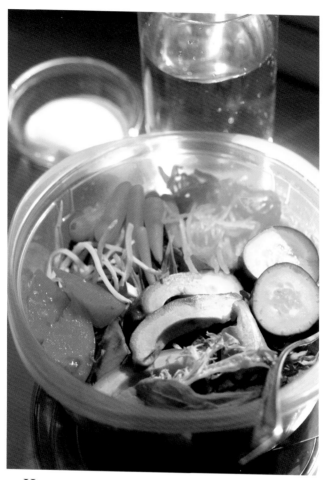

Here you can see I've got some leafy greens, avocado, Romaine lettuce, cucumbers, tomatoes, carrots, baked spaghetti squash. Then of course, I have my dressing of choice on the side.

sprouts, eggplant, cauliflower, collard greens and okra. Cooking increases the energy available from starchy foods such as potatoes, sweet potatoes, beans & peas (but don't eat beans, soybeans and peas *raw.*, *some can be toxic*).

Tempeh (made from whole soybeans) is a great addition to your salad for some additional clean-burning protein and omega-3 fatty acids. It doesn't *"taste like chicken"*, it *"tastes better than chicken"*. You can just slice it up and fry it in some olive oil or coconut oil. On the days that I workout, I'll throw in a small baked potato, sweet potato, baked spaghetti squash, steamed green beans, broccoli, or asparagus in my salad for extra energy.

If you want a change from a salad, make a vegetable stir-fry. Cook your veggies in a pan with some olive oil or coconut oil and a dash of Celtic Sea Salt®, fresh garlic, onion or ginger, only until the veggies begin to soften (about five minutes). The longer you cook most veggies, the more nutrients escape . . . you just want to barely break down their outer cell wall. This makes some veggies absorb better. You can also slice up an avocado and throw it on-top once the veggies have been cooked. Tempeh and low-calorie grains like brown rice, *quinoa* (pronounced keen-wah) and millet also go great with stir-fry. These healthy whole grain / whole food carbs are loaded with fiber and nutrients to balance blood sugar.

Another great idea for lunch is vegetable spaghetti made with spaghetti squash instead of unhealthfully processed noodles. Spaghetti squash is a yellow oblong squash ranging from 1-4lbs. Throw one in the oven and bake at 350 for about 45 minutes and yes you can make this up ahead of time. When the squash is almost finished baking, throw in some fresh broccoli and carrots, red peppers, any veggies you like with some marinara sauce and cook on the stovetop until hot. When the squash is ready, slice it in half, remove the seeds (like a cantaloupe) and rake the pulp of the squash out with a fork. This creates strands of squash just like pasta noodles. It's pretty cool. An option in winter weather would be to add a few handfuls of your favorite fresh vegetables to a can of organic soup and warm on the stovetop for a nutritious warm meal.

Just think for a second how nutritious these foods are for your body. Everything you've eaten so far is easy on your digestive system and essential to your body. Bet you can't say that about your previous diet. So how's your blood sugar, how's your cravings and how 'bout that increased energy. You're gonna love this new lifestyle!

FIFTEEN

Well, we've made it through breakfast, a snack and lunch.

So scarf down another *Raw Crunch® Bar* for a snack on your way home from work and we'll almost be ready to indulge in that *dinner* you've been daydreaming about.

It's time to review our day. You've had your shot of *Greens,* a few pieces of fruit, a *Raw Crunch® Bar,* a pre-made salad, another *Raw Crunch® Bar* and lots of water in between. And now it's almost time for your *dinner meal of choice.* Pretty darn easy, huh? Here's just a few thelpful hints:

1) Keep a jug of purified water in your car at all times! You gotta stay hydrated and keep those toxins

flowing out of your system. If you think you're hungry, evaluate your water intake so far, you may just be low on fluids, so have a big glass of purified water and then evaluate your hunger level.

2) Keep additional fresh fruits around since they act as good filler foods in case of emergency. Their water content and bulk fiber also helps to calm the appetite.

3) If you have a faster metabolism or you ate *dinner* early the night before or had a light *dinner*, you may want to have your first *Raw Crunch® Bar* earlier in the day.

4) If you are having trouble with constipation in the beginning, this is normal since you're not eating so much concentrated food and you may be weaning yourself off of coffee (which increases peristalsis). The *Vitamineral™ Green* usually does the trick, but if the problem lasts for several days, you may need a jumpstart. You may want to consider colon hydrotherapy (a colonic) from a certified colon

therapist when you begin *The Raw Crunch Diet*. All they use is purified water to flush your colon and they are effective and gentle. Stay away from chemical laxatives, we all know their harsh effects on your liver.

SIXTEEN

"Yipee . . . we've made it to *dinner* time!

The main reason why I have chosen *dinner* for the *meal of choice* is because I'm assuming it will consist of some cooked and processed foods, which typically create digestive stress and exhaust the body. So the evening *dinner* is the best time for this to happen.

You may wonder if you can just exchange your *dinner meal of choice* with lunch. Not a good idea . . . besides lowering your energy levels, consuming these non-natural foods early in the day can make your cravings get out of hand. Plus, you will have more time in the day to make bad food choices, as opposed to an evening *meal of choice*. Occasionally, I may replace my *dinner meal of choice* with lunch. Maybe once a month, I've even made breakfast my

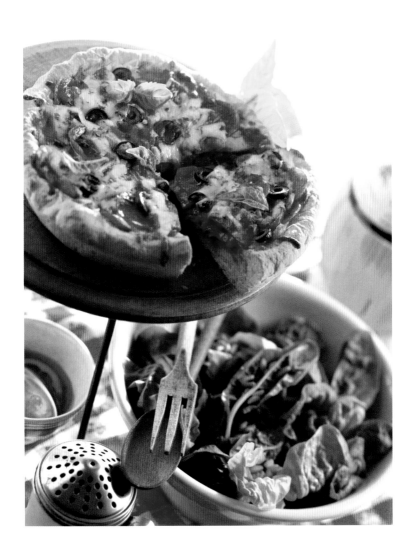

meal of choice. Then the hard part is maintaining the willpower to stay on *The Raw Crunch Diet* for the rest of the day. *"But remember you consume food, you don't let food consume your life, right?"*

My nutrition plan leading up to this daily *dinner* option is crucial for your assured fat loss and radiant health gain. You *must* eat the way that I have outlined up to this point in *The Raw Crunch Diet* during the day, because if your body goes for an extended period of time without food or water, *it will assume there is a shortage* and it will retain every ounce of fluid you've drunk (leaving you bloated) while retaining every morsel of food you've eaten (resulting in weight gain). Now with that said, I can tell you the motivating stuff!

I feel it's important to take some time to draw pleasure from your *dinner* meal rather than shoveling it in while filling your mind with guilt. Food is an entertainment as well as a process of life, shared in a relaxed atmosphere with friends and family. Keep in mind, the first few weeks you'll be day dreaming of really dense foods like cheeseburgers or a big bowl of pasta, but as your body becomes more nourished and your soul becomes more balanced, your *dinner* meal will get progressively healthier. Soon, *dinner* will be so nutritionally satisfying that you won't go bonkers. Your *dinner* will become lighter and lighter ensuring a blissful sleep.   My husband and I take pleasure in preparing a healthy (most of the time) delicious dinner. Yeah, sometimes we fall victim to those late night pizza commercials instead, but we don't over indulge and the majority of our diet is incredibly healthy and nutritious. We even occasionally have a dessert after *dinner*.

This simple act of mindful eating works for us like meditation; food shouldn't be a main contributor or source of mental stress. Diet books are so extreme these days, no wonder we are all so overwhelmed and mentally conflicted when it comes to food. *The Raw Crunch Diet* lifestyle is not about what you can't have, it's about developing a healthy attitude toward food slowly. Enjoy this life and all it has to offer. Oh, and by the way, enjoy your personally selected *dinner* choice!

SEVENTEEN

No need to spend hours in the supermarket.

If Mother Nature created it, chances are, it's much better for us than the more profit driven, synthetic foods that line the grocery shelves. So, hit the produce section first for the majority of your meals, then grab your salad dressing, Tempeh (found in the refrigerated section), some healthy grains (like brown rice, millet or *quinoa*) and whatever you need to make dinner. Make sure you keep extra virgin olive oil and coconut oil on hand for any cooking needs.

For your *Raw Crunch® Bar* and *Vitamineral™ Green*, you can simply go to my website at *www.rawcrunch.com* to order them.

Your Grocery List:

Apples – Peel if they are not organic since the waxed skin contains more pesticides. Consider this fact, peeling also removes some of the vitamins, minerals and fiber, so like I said before - *"try to buy Organic Foods "*.

Apricots – Fresh apricots are not always easy to find since they are only in season in the summer. Have a few dried ones if you enjoy them.

Asparagus

Avocado – I usually buy a few firm avocados and a couple slightly softer (more ripe) ones, not too soft though, then the pulp will be brown instead of tasty and green. The firm ones will be ready to eat in a day if you leave them out on the counter. Refrigerate, if you want them to ripen more slowely.

Bananas

Basil – Fresh basil leaves should always be kept at room temperature. Always finely chop to maximize the flavor.

Beets – Fresh beets are round roots with gray exteriors. Peel the roots and shred or slice for salads.

Blackberries – They're only in season in the early summer, so if you can't find fresh ones, you might find frozen organic blackberries in healthfood stores.

Blueberries – They're only in season in the summer, so if you can't find fresh ones, you might find frozen organic blueberries in health stores.

Broccoli

Brussel Sprouts – They're only in season in the fall, so if you can't find fresh ones, you might find frozen organic brussel sprouts in healthfood stores.

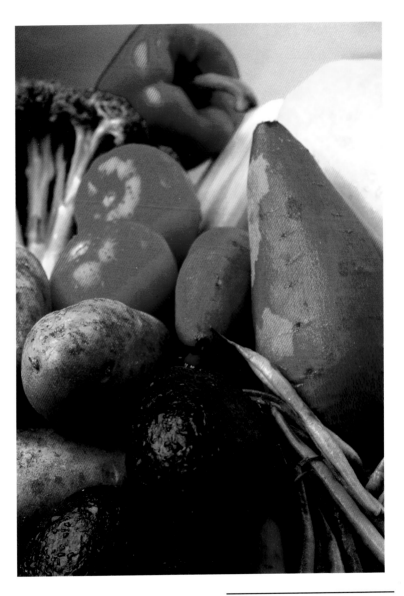

Cabbage

Cantaloupe – Smell the bottom of the cantaloupe, if it smells like fresh cantaloupe, its ripe.

Carrots – The baby ones in the bag are easy enough, right?

Cauliflower

Celery

Cilantro – Always finely chop to maximize it's flavor.

Cucumbers – Peel if they are not organic since the waxed skin contains more pesticides. Unfortunately, as before, peeling also removes some of the vitamins, minerals and fiber, so like I said - *"try to buy Organic Foods".*

Eggplant

Figs – Fresh figs are not always easy to find since they are only in season in the late summer. Have a few dried ones if you enjoy them.

Garlic Root – This is great roasted or sautéed in olive oil and added to any dish.

Ginger Root – Funny shaped tan colored root. Eases an upset stomach if grated and added to warm water. It's also great with steamed veggies.

Grapefruit

Grapes

Green Beans – You can also find frozen organic green beans in healthfood stores.

Honeydew Melon

Kale – It's pretty bitter, but high in calcium if you like it. Not to worry, it's in the *Vitamineral*™ *Green*.

Kiwi – Ripe kiwi should be pretty soft. This fuzzy fruit

should be peeled since the skin is not very tasty.

Lemons/Limes – Extremely cleansing and acts as a mild laxative when added to water.

Lettuce – Anything from Romaine, to Boston, to Arugula, to Watercress (the darker the lettuce, the more nutritious).

Mangos – The softer ones are more ripe. This is one of my favorite fruits!

Okra – They're only in season in the fall, so if you can't find fresh ones, you might find frozen organic okra in healthfood stores.

Onion

Oranges/Tangerines/Nectarines

Papaya – This is a big oblong fruit. If you do not prefer the fresh fruit, they taste great sun dried.

Parsley

Peaches – They're only in season in the summer, so if you can't find fresh ones, you might find frozen organic peaches in health stores. Peel if they are not organic since their fuzzy skin contains more pesticides. Remember, peeling removes some of the vitamins, minerals and fiber, so like I said - *"try to buy Organic Foods"*.

Pears – Peel if they are not organic since their skin contains more pesticides. Again, the peeling issue - *"try to buy Organic Foods"*.

Pineapple – Smell the bottom of the pineapple, if it smells like fresh pineapple, it's ripe. Pineapple contains a digestive enzyme called bromelain which is anti-inflammatory (rinses tissues clean) so I like to have this often for my first fruit in the morning.

Plums – Peel if they are not organic since their skin contains more pesticides. Once again, peeling also removes some of the vitamins, minerals and fiber, so like I said before - *"stick* with Organic Foods".

Pomegranates – Fun to eat in the fall or you can buy the popular antioxidant rich juice to drink with your *Vitamineral™ Green*.

Raspberries – They're only in season in the early summer, so if you can't find fresh ones, you might find frozen organic raspberries in healthfood stores.

Snow Peas – They're only in season in the early spring, so if you can't find fresh ones, you might find frozen organic snow peas in healthfood stores.

Spaghetti Squash – Yellow oblong squash ranging from 1-4lbs. Great replacement for processed pasta noodles, the pulp looks just like strands of spaghetti when baked.

Spinach – Fresh spinach is great in salads and it's also in the *Vitamineral™ Green*

Sprouts – You can grow your own alfalfa sprouts in your house at one-tenth the cost of buying them in the supermarket and you know they are ultra fresh. I put a huge handful in my salad everyday. They're actually really easy to grow and they are ready to eat in just a few days, you don't even need soil or much light to grow them. Most healthfood stores carry spouting trays with simple instructions and all kinds of organic sprouting seeds, from broccoli to bean sprouts. They are a great source of live active enzymes, vitamins and minerals, as well as a very high source of fiber. It took me a while to master *The Raw Crunch Diet*, then I decided I would tackle sprouting, no need to get overwhelmed!

Strawberries – They're only in season in the summer, so if you can't find fresh ones, you might find frozen organic strawberries in healthfood stores.

Sweet Potatoes – Bake in the oven for a sweet and highly nutritious treat. Baked sweet potatoes are great in salads.

Tomatoes– Always keep your tomatoes out on the counter since refrigerated tomatoes get mealy. Once you slice them, they should be refrigerated.

Watermelon – Refreshing and delicious in the summer months.

Yellow Squash/ Zucchini

The Raw Crunch Diet - Daily Recap

MORNING MEAL (see Chapter FIVE)

- 1 Tablespoon *Vitamineral™ Green* mixed in 4-6 ounces of juice.

- Purified Water

- Fresh fruits – Any fruit you like, organic is best!

EARLY AFTERNOON MEAL (see Chapter THIRTEEN)

- *Raw Crunch® Bar* - Choose from Organic Wild Blueberry, Organic Cranberry, Wild Crafted Goji Berry, or Organic Dark Chocolate Chip

- Purified Water

MID-AFTERNOON MEAL (see Chapter FOURTEEN)

- A fresh salad, vegetable stir-fry, or fresh vegetable soup

- Purified water

LATE AFTERNOON MEAL

- Another *Raw Crunch® Bar*

- Purified water

EVENING MEAL (see Chapter SIXTEEN)

- Meal of Choice!

LATE NIGHT SNACK

- Maybe a light desert, some fresh fruit or again *Vitamineral™ Green*

- Purified water

EIGHTEEN

No nutrition program is complete

without regular exercise . . .

However, since 80% of a lean physique is a direct result of your diet, I suggest that you cover this base first! Now that I am on *The Raw Crunch Diet*, I exercise to stay healthy and sculpt my body, rather than over-exercising to loose weight.

The Raw Crunch Diet coupled with regular exercise is a wonderful way to get oxygen and other powerful nutrients into your system. Exercise causes life-supporting oxygen to flow through your veins and accelerates the lymphatic system, sweating and removal of wastes through the skin. We all know how important good blood flow is to the organs and tissues, but proper lymph flow and drainage is also of great importance. The lymphatic system is an important part of the body's immune system and disposes of toxic cellular waste products. This system pumps lymph fluid through the body several times a minute. Accumulation of fluid reduces the amount of oxygen available and can cause swelling in certain areas. Some experts blame lymph accumulation on cellulite. Regular exercise and the cleansing effect of *The Raw Crunch Diet* keep lymph fluid pumping through the body like a free flowing river, without running through rocks or debris. If your diet is loaded with processed, non-natural foods, and you neglect exercise, debris can build up and your system becomes sluggish.

OVER-training (like I use to do in an unsuccessful effort to loose weight) or incorrect form when exercising can sometimes be more detrimental than no exercise at all. If you do a typical aerobic video and throw your body all over the room without constant focused attention to proper form, you are often doing more harm than good. The same applies in the gym, working out with weights. See, strength training naturally causes microscopic tears in your muscle membrane allowing muscles to grow back stronger, and that is normal (as weird as it sounds). However, if your form and body alignment is not correct, those tissues will take longer to heal, producing more cellular waste. In worst cases, those muscles will grow back in the wrong alignment at the expense of your body balance.

Whenever your body undergoes trauma as with these microscopic muscle tears, it sends blood and fluid to those areas to heal the tissues. This causes the *puffiness*, and it is one of the main reasons people get so discouraged when beginning a training regimen. As a fitness competitor, I would have to stop all leg training ten (10) days before my competitions, to reduce fluid build-up in my legs. Otherwise, I would have *a smooth look* rather than defined leg muscles. Like most body-builders and fitness

*Here I am performing a **Single Leg Lunge** which puts special emphasis on my thighs and booty , but due to the*

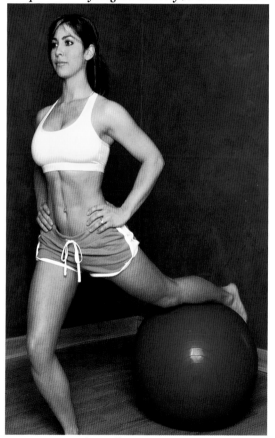

*instability of the **Body Ball**, I'm also working my abdominals and lower back , as well as the tiny stabilizing muscles surrounding my knees and ankles .*

competitors, I would also try and keep my legs up, above my heart, as long as possible throughout the day prior to my competition to reduce fluid collection. Those were the days prior to my development of *The Raw Crunch Diet* and *The Raw Crunch Workout*™ (DVD). Now my tissues always remain healthy with proper flow and drainage.

The focused *Raw Crunch Workout*™ is amazing for stretching and lengthening my body, rather than tightening and shortening the body like conventional body-sculpting workouts. In the *Workout*™ DVD, I provide you with extra attention to breathing, body alignment, and technique, further helping to oxygenate your cells and flush your tissues clean. This type of focused training and deep breathing boosts your ability to feel what's going on inside your body. This body awareness not only detects whether your hamstrings or hips are tight, but also whether your stomach is already full.

The instability of the Body Ball in this Hamstring Curl exercise puts special emphasis on my hamstring muscles , while automatically working

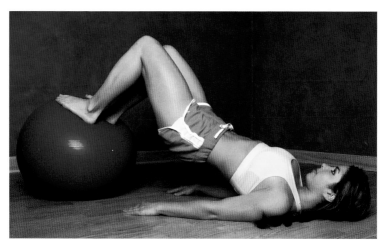

my trunk stabilizing muscles which include the abdominals , lower back and booty in one coordinated movement .

NINETEEN

Just some final thoughts . . .

Warm Celtic Sea Salt® baths are great to further relax your muscles as well as enhance a sound sleep. The healthy nutrients in the salt are absorbed through your tissues to help heal the muscles while the sodium helps pull excess fluid out of the tissues. In addition, to their dietary Celtic Sea Salt®, *www.celtic-seasalt.com* also offers an ultra-healing Celtic Sea Salt® for baths. Don't forget to mention *The Raw Crunch Diet* and receive a 55% member-discount on your first order of these two products. Regular deep tissue massage also increases the nourishing oxygen and blood supply to your tissues while helping to eliminate metabolic wastes and improves lymphatic flow.

For skincare, I use organic, raw coconut oil on my

body, which has a heating effect to further stimulate circulation. It gives my skin a lustrous, healthy glow! Coconut oil also contains natural protective antioxidants, which penetrate into the deeper layers of the skin to strengthen the underlying tissues. I try not to put anything on my skin that I wouldn't eat since the skin is your largest organ. The only problem is *my doggies* love the taste so they try constantly to lick it off my legs. Hey, at least it's good for them.

Coconut oil is the healthiest oil to cook with. Yes it's a saturated fat, but coconut oil is made-up of medium chained fatty acids, which are smaller than other saturated fats and digest VERY QUICKLY for use as an energy source. They do not have time to stick to your hips or clog your arteries. The best source of organic, raw coconut oil is by far *Coco in the Raw.* Also on-line, you can find it along with additional information on this overlooked gift of nature at *www.bodyfriendlyprovisions.com.*

The environment, as well as the nutritional environment that you provide for your body has a direct effect on your health. With our cooperation in supplying our body with essential nutrients and proper hydration, we are equipped to combat the onset of illness and effectively maintain a state of well-being.

And the last element . . . to gain further self-confidence and how to explain this diet to others while confidently answering their uninformed objections or those pesky questions your friends might ask about how *The Raw Crunch Diet* actually works . . . just quick read this book over once again . . . the answers are all there!

In Strong Health,

 Kathy

To Purchase your

* *Raw Crunch® Bars*
* *Vitamineral™ Green*
* *Liver Rescue III + ™*

and

The Raw Crunch Workout™ DVD

Go to my website:

www.rawcrunch.com

Acknowledgment

My heartfelt gratitude goes to Dr. Jameth Sheridan (N.D.) of *HealthForce Nutritionals*, who reviewed my entire book. His valuable contributions are found throughout my efforts and he is a virtual encyclopedia of knowledge on Diet, Holistic Health, Raw Foods, Veganism, and Nutritional Supplements. His feedback elevated *The Raw Crunch Diet* to a whole new level.

Dedication

I dedicate this book to my loving family and especially to my Grandfather, who taught me to "Stop to smell the flowers", told me that "A college education doesn't necessarily make you smarter, it just gives you the GOLDEN opportunity to express your ignorance", and as he dropped my brother and I off at the bus stop everyday he would tell us to "Have a good day, and if you can't have a good day, [we would smile and say *I know, I know*] *make it miserable for everyone else*". I love you Grandpa.

About the Author
Kathy Feldman

Kathy has twelve years of experience in the fields of corrective and high performance exercise health and nutrition. An honors graduate from East Carolina University, Kathy has a Bachelors of Science degree in Cellular Biology. Following college she became a successful National Fitness America competitor and sports model. Recently, Kathy has founded Body Engineering, Inc. with the objective of establishing a company to manufacture her ultimate health food formula, trademarked as ***Raw Crunch® Bars***. In addition to ***The Raw Crunch Diet*** , Kathy has produced the ***Raw Crunch Workout*** ™ ***DVD*** adding the final aspect to her wellness concept. To Kathy there is nothing more rewarding than helping someone to realize their own potential. Her ultimate objective is to lead by example, working in a field that she loves and contributing to the quality of life of others.

And thirdly, it is doable, for life! *The Raw Crunch Diet* program is easy to follow. You will eat good tasting food. It allows for flexibility and individual choices – it is built right in. It is *not* an all or nothing approach. What good is a diet that is not sustainable? *The Raw Crunch Diet* allows you success, while being able to live your life (leaner and healthier).

If you want to lose fat, get healthier, and even eat in a way that is more compassionate and better for the planet, then *The Raw Crunch Diet* is for you!"

- *Jameth Sheridan, N.D.*
- *Nutritional Research Scientist*
  www.rawfoodresearch.com

"*Raw Crunch*® *Bars* have all the major eye vitamins proven to be effective in combating macular degeneration. The Omega-3 fatty acids also in *Raw Crunch*® *Bars* help prevent dry eye symptoms and are good for your cardiovascular health.

I eat two *Raw Crunch® Bars* every day!"

- Jonathan D. Christenbury, M.D. - Medical Director

Christenbury Eye Center - Charlotte, N.C.

www.christenbury.com

"Though I was aware of all the health benefits of *raw food* and the *Raw Crunch® Bars*, I was amazed at how great they taste. The New Jersey Women and AIDS Network provides *Raw Crunch® Bars* as a healthy snack alternative to the HIV+ Women they provide services to. Never before have I seen the women we work with eagerly consume such a healthy product.

Thanks, Kathy."

- Elizabeth Roberts - Health Education Specialist

New Jersey Women and AIDS Network

www.njwan.org

"When I read the ingredients in the *Raw Crunch® Bars* I was very surprised that they were truly raw and seemed very 'pure'. Usually most of the bars, even though they say they are *raw*, have some kind of ingredients that make you doubt it, like grains or sweeteners, etc. My next thought was that they could not possibly taste very good, as looking at the ingredients there seemed to be just all-organic nuts, seeds, fruit, and a little honey. Being *raw* for 14 years, I was excited that they appeared 100% *raw*, but being a gourmet *raw food chef* I was skeptical about the taste. Well, I was shocked that they were so good! The flavor of these bars are incredible! I am so excited to finally have a fast, healthy, great tasting, *all raw bar* to promote to my clients!

Whether you're an athlete, *raw fooder* or just want to take a healthy snack with you during the work day, the *Raw Crunch® Bar* is the best I've seen so far!"

- Alissa Cohen, Raw Food Chef & Educator
www.alissacohen.com

"I have used your *Raw Crunch® Bars* with my patients and myself for the past few months. There are no words that can express what a joy it is to be able to offer a bar that is not only extremely good for you but, also has a taste that makes you want more. This is truly a work of love and not money. My patients are amazed at being able to lose weight and still have something so satisfying to eat.

Thank you again, Kathy, for this wonderful food."

- Dr. Rebecca McCall, Charlotte, NC